FUNCTIONAL APPROACH TO PSYCHIATRIC TREATMENT

A PRACTICAL GUIDE FOR MENTAL HEALTH PROFESSIONALS

© **Copyright 2024 - All rights reserved.**

The content contained within this book may not be reproduced, duplicated or transmitted without direct written permission from the author or the publisher.

Under no circumstances will any blame or legal responsibility be held against the publisher, or author, for any damages, reparation, or monetary loss due to the information contained within this book. Either directly or indirectly.

Legal Notice:

This book is copyright protected. This book is only for personal use. You cannot amend, distribute, sell, use, quote or paraphrase any part, or the content within this book, without the consent of the author or publisher.

Disclaimer Notice:

Please note the information contained within this document is for educational and entertainment purposes only. All effort has been executed to present accurate, up to date, and reliable, complete information. No warranties of any kind are declared or implied. Readers acknowledge that the author is not engaging in the rendering of legal, financial, medical or professional advice. The content within this book has been derived from various sources. Please consult a licensed professional before attempting any techniques outlined in this book.

By reading this document, the reader agrees that under no circumstances is the author responsible for any losses, direct or indirect, which are incurred as a result of the use of information contained within this document, including, but not limited to, — errors, omissions, or inaccuracies.

DESCRIPTION 4

INTRODUCTION 6

CHAPTER 1: CORE PRINCIPLES OF FUNCTIONAL PSYCHIATRY 11

CHAPTER 2: FUNCTIONAL DIAGNOSTIC APPROACHES IN PSYCHIATRY 23

CHAPTER 3: DEVELOPING AN INTEGRATIVE TREATMENT PLAN 34

CHAPTER 4: INTEGRATING THERAPEUTIC TECHNIQUES IN FUNCTIONAL PSYCHIATRY 45

CHAPTER 5: IMPLEMENTING FUNCTIONAL PSYCHIATRY IN CLINICAL PRACTICE 54

CONCLUSION 64

Description

Are you a mental health professional looking to move beyond symptom management and offer transformative, root-cause-focused care?

For too long, psychiatry has been driven by a narrow focus on managing symptoms through medication and brief interventions. But what if there was a way to address mental health holistically, by looking at the mind, body, and environment as a whole? *Functional Approach to Psychiatric Treatment: A Practical Guide for Mental Health Professionals* introduces you to a comprehensive, integrative approach that goes beyond traditional psychiatry, aiming to identify and address the underlying causes of mental health conditions.

In this essential guide, you'll discover how functional psychiatry combines the best of traditional mental health treatment with the latest insights in nutrition, lifestyle medicine, and mind-body practices, empowering both you and your patients to achieve sustainable mental wellness. You will learn how to:

- **Uncover root causes** of psychiatric symptoms, from biochemical imbalances and inflammation to lifestyle factors, transforming the way you understand and treat mental health.

- **Create personalized, holistic treatment plans** that integrate diet, exercise, sleep, and stress management—foundations that support lasting mental health.

- **Incorporate effective therapeutic techniques** like cognitive-behavioral therapy (CBT), mindfulness, and biofeedback to complement functional treatments and foster resilience.

- **Collaborate with multidisciplinary professionals** such as nutritionists, physical therapists, and mindfulness practitioners to provide well-rounded, patient-centered care.

- **Engage patients in their own healing journey**, building trust and motivation by helping them understand the benefits of a functional approach.

Packed with practical tools, case studies, and actionable steps, *Functional Approach to Psychiatric Treatment* provides a roadmap for integrating this holistic model into your practice. Whether you're new to functional psychiatry or looking to deepen your skills, this book offers the knowledge and strategies to create real, lasting improvements for your patients.

Don't let outdated treatment models hold you back. Take the first step toward transforming your practice with *Functional Approach to Psychiatric Treatment* and discover the power of a truly holistic approach to mental health.

Introduction

Traditional psychiatry, while effective for many, often relies on symptom management and medication, leaving some patients feeling stuck or underserved. Many struggle with recurring mental health symptoms, despite standard treatments, and find that their broader health concerns—diet, lifestyle, physical symptoms—are rarely addressed in conventional settings. These limitations have created a demand for an approach that goes beyond symptom suppression.

Functional psychiatry addresses these challenges by shifting the focus to the underlying causes of mental health issues, considering not only the brain but also the body and lifestyle factors that contribute to emotional and cognitive health. As patients increasingly seek holistic, integrative care, the need for functional psychiatry becomes clear: it's an approach that treats the whole person, emphasizing wellness and resilience over quick fixes. This model aims to meet patients' needs on every level, from physical to emotional, setting the stage for more sustainable mental health care.

Functional psychiatry is an integrative approach that looks beyond symptoms to address the root causes of mental health conditions. Unlike traditional models, which often focus on managing symptoms through medication, functional psychiatry seeks to uncover and treat the underlying factors that may be driving mental health challenges. This approach considers **physical, psychological, and environmental influences**, including genetics, diet, lifestyle, and trauma history, to create a complete understanding of each patient's health.

Where traditional psychiatry might focus on diagnosing and treating isolated symptoms, functional psychiatry emphasizes **root-cause analysis and interconnected systems**. It examines how different aspects of a patient's health—such as their immune function, gut health, and stress levels—interact and impact mental well-being. The goal is not only to alleviate symptoms but to build long-term mental wellness and resilience, empowering patients with tools to manage their health comprehensively.

Functional psychiatry is guided by principles that differentiate it from other mental health approaches, making it uniquely suited to addressing complex mental health needs.

- **Mind-Body Connection**: Functional psychiatry is rooted in the belief that mental and physical health are deeply interconnected. Issues like inflammation, nutrient deficiencies, and hormonal imbalances can significantly impact mood and cognitive function. This model recognizes that the brain and body operate as a cohesive unit, with physical imbalances often manifesting as mental health symptoms.

- **Root-Cause Analysis**: Instead of merely treating symptoms, functional psychiatry aims to uncover and address the underlying causes of mental health issues. Practitioners conduct in-depth assessments to identify contributors such as lifestyle factors, genetics, and biochemical imbalances, focusing on sustainable solutions rather than temporary fixes.

- **Individualized, Patient-Centered Care**: Each patient's journey and health profile are unique, so functional psychiatry places a strong emphasis on customized treatment. Practitioners develop individualized plans that account for a patient's lifestyle, genetics, and health history, creating a plan that's tailored to each person's specific needs.

- **Integrative and Collaborative Approach**: Functional psychiatry often involves collaboration with other health professionals, such as nutritionists, physical therapists, and mindfulness practitioners. This interdisciplinary approach ensures that patients receive comprehensive care that addresses all aspects of their well-being.

Functional psychiatry can benefit a broad range of patients, particularly those who have found traditional psychiatric treatments insufficient or who seek a more comprehensive approach to mental health.

- **Patients with Chronic Mental Health Conditions**: Those dealing with recurring issues like depression, anxiety, or mood instability that persist despite traditional treatments often find functional psychiatry effective in addressing these complex conditions.

- **Individuals with Physical and Mental Health Overlaps**: Patients experiencing both mental and physical symptoms, such as chronic fatigue or digestive issues alongside mood disorders, can benefit from the integrative approach of functional psychiatry, which addresses these interconnected health issues.

- **Those Seeking Holistic Care**: Patients who prefer a root-cause approach and wish to understand the broader factors affecting their mental health often find functional psychiatry aligns well with their desire for comprehensive care.

This book is designed to guide you through the essential elements of functional psychiatry, from foundational principles to practical implementation. Each chapter builds on the last, creating a cohesive understanding of this approach:

- **Chapter 1** explores the core principles of functional psychiatry, offering a foundation for understanding its unique approach and distinctions from traditional psychiatry.

- **Chapter 2** covers diagnostic tools and assessment methods that help identify the root causes of mental health conditions, including lifestyle, nutritional, and biological factors.

- **Chapter 3** provides a comprehensive guide to creating personalized treatment plans that integrate diet, sleep, movement, and stress management, essential components for mental wellness.

- **Chapter 4** delves into therapeutic techniques that complement functional psychiatry, such as CBT, mindfulness, and biofeedback, and explains how to incorporate these methods into a holistic treatment plan.

- **Chapter 5** offers practical guidance for implementing functional psychiatry in clinical practice, focusing on patient communication, building a support network, and creating a collaborative, resource-rich environment.

- **Conclusion** reflects on the future of functional psychiatry, encouraging continued learning and adaptation as the field evolves.

This structure provides a step-by-step approach to understanding and applying functional psychiatry in your practice, empowering you to make a lasting difference in the lives of your patients.

Functional psychiatry represents a transformative approach to mental health care, one that challenges practitioners to think beyond symptoms and engage with the full complexity of each patient's health. This book invites you to explore functional psychiatry with an open mind, recognizing the potential for this model to create deeper, more sustainable healing.

As you move through these pages, consider each concept and strategy as a tool for **patient-centered care**—an approach that respects the unique experiences and needs of each individual. By adopting functional psychiatry, you have the opportunity to offer patients a path to true wellness, equipping them with the knowledge and support they need to thrive.

The functional approach has the power to transform not only patient outcomes but also the practice of psychiatry itself, fostering a field that is as holistic as it is effective.

Chapter 1: Core Principles of Functional Psychiatry

"Healing is a matter of time, but it is sometimes also a matter of opportunity."
— *Hippocrates*

A young woman in her late twenties had cycled through nearly every available medication for anxiety and depression, each new prescription offering only a temporary respite. With no clear answers beyond more symptom-masking drugs, she began to question whether her mental health could be fully restored. When her care shifted to a functional approach, her treatment expanded from focusing solely on her brain to exploring underlying factors in her body, lifestyle, and environment. Her healing was no longer simply a matter of suppressing symptoms but of addressing root causes—a transformative shift that gradually unlocked real, sustainable mental well-being.

This chapter lays the groundwork for understanding the fundamental differences between traditional and functional psychiatry. You'll learn why functional psychiatry's patient-centered, holistic approach is essential for addressing root causes rather than symptoms alone. Core principles such as the mind-body connection and root-cause analysis form the foundation of this approach, offering a framework that integrates lifestyle factors, biological markers, and mental health for more comprehensive, lasting treatment outcomes.

Functional Psychiatry vs. Traditional Psychiatry

In psychiatry, traditional and functional approaches represent two distinct frameworks for addressing mental health. Traditional psychiatry generally focuses on diagnosing symptoms and alleviating them through medications or therapeutic techniques. While effective in symptom reduction, it often bypasses deeper biological, lifestyle, and environmental contributors. **Functional psychiatry**, however, seeks to address these root causes, emphasizing a **holistic approach** that views mental health as interconnected with overall physical well-being. This section will explore these approaches, highlighting the core distinctions that make functional psychiatry a comprehensive alternative for those seeking sustainable mental health solutions.

Traditional psychiatry has long been guided by a **symptom-management model**, focusing on identifying symptoms that match specific psychiatric disorders and selecting medications to alleviate them. **Pharmacotherapy** is often the primary tool, used to manage conditions like depression, anxiety, bipolar disorder, and schizophrenia. In this model, symptoms are seen as manifestations of imbalances within the brain's neurochemistry. Prescribing medications to correct these imbalances is standard, supported by therapeutic modalities like cognitive-behavioral therapy (CBT) to help patients cope with their conditions. Traditional psychiatry has brought significant relief to many individuals and remains indispensable for crisis situations and severe disorders. However, it frequently overlooks **underlying factors**—such as nutrition, sleep patterns, chronic stress, and physical health—that can perpetuate or exacerbate mental health conditions.

Functional psychiatry, by contrast, operates on the belief that mental health issues are rarely isolated to the mind alone. It assumes that **underlying causes**—including inflammation, hormonal imbalances, nutritional deficiencies, and lifestyle stressors—can drive psychiatric symptoms. Rather than focusing on a single organ (the brain), functional psychiatry views the body as an interconnected system. Practitioners aim to create personalized treatment plans that address each patient's unique physiological, environmental, and lifestyle factors. This approach considers the **mind-body connection**, recognizing that mental health symptoms may signal broader imbalances within the body. For example, gut health has been shown to influence mood and cognition, leading functional psychiatrists to address digestive health as part of treatment for mood disorders.

Key differences between the two approaches reveal the **broader scope** of functional psychiatry. Traditional psychiatry often centers on **symptom suppression** through medication, seeking immediate relief for patients. Functional psychiatry, however, emphasizes **root-cause treatment**, which involves identifying the specific factors driving mental health issues and addressing them directly. While traditional psychiatry may prioritize medications to "correct" brain chemistry, functional psychiatry uses **holistic interventions** such as nutritional counseling, stress management techniques, sleep optimization, and exercise routines, often incorporating these elements alongside or instead of pharmaceuticals. **Collaborative care** is also a hallmark of functional psychiatry, which may involve coordination with other specialists, like nutritionists, physical therapists, or endocrinologists, to create a comprehensive treatment plan.

Consider a patient suffering from chronic depression who, after years of various medications, found little improvement in her overall well-being. Under a functional psychiatry approach, her treatment was expanded to include dietary adjustments, sleep tracking, and stress-reduction techniques. Over time, these targeted interventions not only lifted her depressive symptoms but also improved her overall quality of life. Functional psychiatry's **integrative, personalized approach** offered her sustainable relief by addressing root causes rather than masking symptoms. This case highlights the potential for **lasting improvement** through functional psychiatry, distinguishing it from the more narrowly focused methods of traditional psychiatry.

Key Principles of Functional Psychiatry

Functional psychiatry is founded on principles that seek to identify and address the underlying contributors to mental health conditions, looking beyond symptoms to understand the full context of an individual's health. Key to this approach is the recognition that mental health is not isolated from physical health; rather, it is deeply influenced by lifestyle, environmental, and physiological factors. This section covers three essential principles of functional psychiatry: the **mind-body connection**, **root-cause analysis**, and the **integrative approach**. Together, these principles form the backbone of a comprehensive, patient-centered approach that aims for sustainable mental health outcomes.

Mind-Body Connection

A foundational principle of functional psychiatry is the understanding that the mind and body are interconnected systems, each profoundly influencing the other. **Mental health cannot be fully understood or treated in isolation from physical health.** Evidence has shown that physiological factors—such as gut health, hormone balance, and inflammatory processes—can significantly impact mood regulation, cognitive function, and overall mental well-being. For instance, the gut-brain axis, a bi-directional communication pathway between the gastrointestinal tract and the brain, plays a critical role in mood and cognition. Disruptions in gut health, such as imbalances in gut bacteria, can lead to inflammation and release neuroactive compounds that affect the brain, potentially contributing to anxiety, depression, and cognitive decline.

Hormones also play a significant role in this connection. Imbalances in hormones like cortisol, thyroid hormones, and sex hormones (such as estrogen and testosterone) can manifest as mental health symptoms, including fatigue, mood swings, and cognitive difficulties. Elevated cortisol, often a result of chronic stress, can lead to anxiety and depression by disrupting neurotransmitter function and causing inflammation in the brain. Functional psychiatry considers these hormonal influences and integrates methods to regulate them, such as stress management practices, lifestyle adjustments, and dietary interventions.

Inflammation is another physical factor closely tied to mental health. Chronic inflammation in the body can increase the risk of mood disorders and impair cognitive function. Functional psychiatry approaches inflammation by addressing its sources, such as poor diet, lack of exercise, and environmental toxins, to promote mental and physical health holistically. By viewing mental health through the lens of the **mind-body connection**, functional psychiatry offers a comprehensive approach that acknowledges and treats the biological, psychological, and lifestyle factors influencing a patient's well-being.

Root-Cause Analysis

In traditional psychiatry, the focus often remains on identifying symptoms and assigning diagnoses that lead to treatment with medication or therapy. **Root-cause analysis**, however, is central to functional psychiatry, which seeks to understand what is driving these symptoms in the first place. This process involves exploring beyond surface symptoms to uncover potential **underlying factors** such as inflammation, nutrient deficiencies, chronic stress, and hormonal imbalances. Rather than asking, "How can we manage this symptom?" functional psychiatry asks, "What is causing this symptom to appear?"

For example, a patient presenting with persistent fatigue and low mood may be prescribed an antidepressant in a traditional setting. However, root-cause analysis in functional psychiatry would investigate whether the patient has underlying issues, such as hypothyroidism, anemia, or a Vitamin D deficiency. Correcting these root causes could eliminate the need for antidepressants, providing a more sustainable and personalized solution. **Identifying nutrient deficiencies** is a frequent focus of root-cause analysis, as imbalances in vitamins and minerals—like B vitamins, magnesium, and omega-3 fatty acids—are known to impact mood and brain function. Functional psychiatry assesses these deficiencies and integrates dietary or supplemental recommendations as part of treatment.

Another key component of root-cause analysis is evaluating lifestyle factors. Chronic stress, for instance, can contribute to anxiety and depression by continually elevating cortisol levels and impairing the body's ability to return to a state of balance. Functional psychiatry addresses this by incorporating stress management techniques, sleep optimization, and regular physical activity into the treatment plan. Root-cause analysis thus enables practitioners to craft treatments tailored to the individual, aiming for long-term improvements rather than temporary symptom relief.

Integrative Approach

Functional psychiatry's **integrative approach** addresses mental health by considering the many factors that contribute to an individual's well-being. This approach views mental health within a broader ecosystem that includes physical, psychological, environmental, and social dimensions. Functional psychiatrists create treatment plans that encompass **lifestyle adjustments, nutritional guidance, and environmental considerations**. For instance, if a patient's depression is exacerbated by poor diet and lack of exercise, the integrative approach would incorporate nutritional improvements and an exercise regimen into their care plan.

Functional psychiatry often involves **collaborative care**, where psychiatrists work alongside other health professionals, including nutritionists, physical therapists, and endocrinologists, to develop a comprehensive treatment plan. This collaborative model enhances the effectiveness of treatment by addressing various health factors simultaneously. For example, a nutritionist might work with a psychiatrist to correct dietary issues contributing to a patient's mood disorder, or a physical therapist might assist in designing an exercise program to improve mental health outcomes. This multidisciplinary approach ensures that patients receive **holistic care** that addresses all aspects of their health.

Functional psychiatry's key principles—the mind-body connection, root-cause analysis, and integrative approach—offer a paradigm shift from traditional models, aiming to treat the whole person rather than isolated symptoms. This comprehensive, patient-centered framework sets the stage for a more sustainable and effective path to mental well-being.

The Role of Lifestyle in Mental Health

Functional psychiatry places significant emphasis on lifestyle factors as core components of mental health. Unlike traditional models, which may focus predominantly on symptom management through medication, functional psychiatry views mental health as closely interconnected with daily habits and biological needs. This section highlights the roles of **diet and nutrition**, **exercise and physical activity**, **sleep**, and **stress management** in mental well-being, underscoring how addressing these elements can lead to more sustainable mental health outcomes.

Diet and Nutrition

Diet plays a critical role in mental health, as the brain relies on a consistent supply of essential nutrients to maintain optimal function. Nutritional deficiencies and imbalanced diets can lead to mood disorders, cognitive impairments, and other mental health issues. **Omega-3 fatty acids**, for example, are known for their anti-inflammatory properties and are crucial for brain health, impacting mood regulation and cognitive function. Research has linked omega-3 deficiencies to higher rates of depression and anxiety, emphasizing the importance of a diet rich in fatty fish, flaxseeds, and walnuts. **B vitamins**, particularly B12 and folate, are also essential for cognitive health and the production of neurotransmitters like serotonin and dopamine, which regulate mood and motivation. Low levels of B vitamins can contribute to depressive symptoms and fatigue, highlighting the importance of sources like leafy greens, eggs, and legumes in one's diet.

Additionally, **blood sugar regulation** is a key factor in maintaining mood stability. Diets high in refined sugars and processed carbohydrates can cause spikes and crashes in blood sugar levels, leading to irritability, anxiety, and depressive symptoms. For instance, a patient suffering from mood swings and irritability saw improvements after adjusting her diet to include more whole foods, lean proteins, and complex carbohydrates. By stabilizing her blood sugar levels, she experienced fewer mood fluctuations and improved mental clarity. This case underscores the importance of balanced nutrition in maintaining stable mood and energy levels.

Exercise and Physical Activity

Regular physical activity has been shown to have numerous benefits for mental health, impacting both **mood and cognitive function**. Physical exercise stimulates the release of endorphins, dopamine, and serotonin—neurotransmitters associated with pleasure, motivation, and mood regulation. Aerobic exercises, like running, swimming, and cycling, are particularly effective for releasing these "feel-good" chemicals and enhancing mood. Studies have shown that consistent aerobic activity can reduce symptoms of depression and anxiety, even matching the efficacy of some antidepressant medications in certain cases.

Strength training also has notable benefits for mental health, helping reduce symptoms of anxiety and improve resilience to stress. This type of exercise enhances physical strength, which can also boost self-esteem and body confidence, factors known to contribute to a positive self-image. A functional psychiatry approach may incorporate tailored exercise routines into treatment plans, recognizing that physical health is inseparable from mental well-being. Whether through structured workouts or recreational activities, maintaining a consistent exercise routine can significantly improve mood stability and overall mental clarity.

Sleep

Sleep is foundational to mental health, yet sleep disturbances are common among individuals with psychiatric disorders. Inadequate or poor-quality sleep can lead to irritability, poor concentration, and increased vulnerability to stress, contributing to a cycle of mental health decline. During sleep, the brain processes emotional experiences, consolidates memories, and repairs cellular damage, making restful sleep crucial for cognitive and emotional resilience.

Sleep issues, such as insomnia and sleep apnea, are often present in mood disorders like depression and anxiety. Functional psychiatry addresses sleep by encouraging **sleep optimization techniques** to improve sleep quality and duration. Simple strategies such as maintaining a consistent sleep schedule, limiting caffeine intake in the afternoon, and creating a calm, dark bedroom environment can significantly improve sleep patterns. Additionally, the practice of **sleep hygiene**—which includes winding down before bed, avoiding screen time, and relaxing activities like reading or meditation—can help reduce insomnia and enhance sleep quality. By prioritizing restorative sleep, functional psychiatry promotes a foundation for mental resilience and improved mood.

Stress Management

Chronic stress is a major contributor to mental health issues, with physiological effects that can lead to mood disorders, anxiety, and cognitive impairment. Prolonged stress raises cortisol levels, which, if left unchecked, can damage the hippocampus (responsible for memory and learning) and disrupt neurotransmitter balance. Functional psychiatry recognizes that managing stress is essential for maintaining mental health and incorporates **stress-reduction techniques** as part of a holistic treatment approach.

Effective stress management practices include **mindfulness, meditation, and breathing exercises**, all of which have been shown to lower cortisol levels and enhance mental clarity. Mindfulness helps individuals stay grounded in the present, reducing rumination and emotional reactivity. Meditation practices, even when practiced briefly each day, can improve attention, mood stability, and overall stress resilience. Deep breathing exercises activate the body's relaxation response, helping to alleviate acute stress and anxiety. By incorporating these methods, functional psychiatry provides tools for patients to better manage stress and its impact on mental health.

Integrating Lifestyle Factors in Functional Psychiatry

The role of lifestyle factors in mental health is central to functional psychiatry's comprehensive, patient-centered approach. By addressing diet, physical activity, sleep, and stress management, functional psychiatry equips patients with sustainable tools to improve and maintain mental health. Each of these lifestyle elements plays a unique role in the overall picture of well-being, and their integration in treatment plans offers a pathway to lasting mental resilience and health stability.

Key Takeaways

Functional psychiatry provides a holistic framework for mental health care, prioritizing **root-cause identification** over mere symptom management. The **mind-body connection** is essential, as physical health directly influences mental well-being. **Lifestyle factors** like diet, exercise, and sleep significantly impact mental health and are integral to treatment planning. By considering these elements, functional psychiatry offers a comprehensive approach that supports sustainable mental wellness and resilience.

Action Step: Reflect on a lifestyle factor—such as sleep, diet, or exercise—that you've observed affecting mental health in your patients or yourself.

Call to Action: Continue to the next chapter to dive deeper into the functional diagnostic process and learn practical steps for implementing this approach.

Chapter 2: Functional Diagnostic Approaches in Psychiatry

"Diagnosis is not the end, but the beginning of practice."
— Martin H. Fischer

A young man in his thirties, who had been treated for chronic anxiety and fatigue with multiple medications over several years, struggled with ongoing symptoms despite extensive traditional evaluations. Yet, no standard tests revealed why he still felt exhausted and unfocused. A shift to a **functional diagnostic approach** changed everything. By examining his inflammatory markers and nutritional profile, his care team discovered a severe Vitamin D deficiency and high levels of systemic inflammation. Addressing these root causes brought him a level of relief he hadn't experienced in years, underscoring how powerful a comprehensive, functional diagnostic approach can be for patients facing unresolved symptoms.

This chapter provides a detailed framework for a functional approach to psychiatric diagnosis, showing how this method goes beyond conventional evaluations. We'll discuss the **importance of a holistic diagnostic perspective** that incorporates biological markers, lifestyle factors, and the gut-brain connection. Key diagnostic tools and insights will be introduced, offering practical steps to help mental health professionals implement functional diagnostic methods in their practice to uncover and address underlying causes of psychiatric symptoms.

Comprehensive Functional Assessment

A comprehensive functional assessment in psychiatry is about looking at the whole picture—not just symptoms but the interconnected physical, mental, and lifestyle factors that influence mental health. Traditional assessments may stop at diagnosis, focusing primarily on psychiatric symptoms and immediate treatments. Functional psychiatry, however, recognizes that lasting mental health improvement requires a deep understanding of the unique biological, psychological, and environmental contributors to a patient's condition. This section outlines the components of a thorough functional assessment, which extends beyond the boundaries of traditional evaluations to identify the root causes driving psychiatric symptoms.

Holistic Evaluation

A functional assessment starts with a **holistic evaluation** that considers the patient's full health history, examining genetic predispositions, lifestyle choices, and environmental exposures. Understanding these elements is crucial because mental health is rarely isolated from other bodily systems. For example, a patient's family history of autoimmune disorders may raise suspicion of underlying inflammatory processes, which could be contributing to symptoms of depression or anxiety. Lifestyle factors, such as diet, exercise habits, and sleep patterns, provide essential clues. Environmental exposures, including chronic stress or exposure to toxins, can also shape mental health outcomes over time. By thoroughly exploring these aspects, practitioners can better understand each patient's vulnerabilities and the potential underlying contributors to their symptoms. This wide-ranging view is foundational in functional psychiatry, where the goal is not simply to alleviate symptoms but to address the underlying factors that keep these symptoms alive.

Physical Health Markers

Physical health markers play a central role in functional assessments, as physical imbalances often influence mental states. Key markers include **inflammatory markers** like C-reactive protein (CRP), which can indicate systemic inflammation linked to mood disorders. Thyroid function tests are also critical, as thyroid imbalances—often overlooked in traditional psychiatric evaluations—can lead to symptoms of depression, fatigue, and anxiety. Hormonal levels, such as cortisol and sex hormones (e.g., estrogen, testosterone), also provide insights. Elevated cortisol levels, often associated with chronic stress, can disrupt sleep, elevate anxiety, and lower resilience to stress. By assessing these markers, practitioners gain a clearer view of how physical health may be contributing to or exacerbating mental health symptoms.

Mental Health History

Understanding a patient's **psychiatric history** is essential for developing a nuanced treatment plan. A detailed history reveals past diagnoses, treatment responses, and any previous experiences with medications or therapies. For instance, a patient's history of poor responses to certain medications may suggest that their symptoms stem from non-psychiatric sources, such as metabolic or hormonal issues. Trauma history is also a critical element, as unresolved trauma can significantly impact brain function, stress resilience, and emotional regulation. Functional psychiatry examines this history to identify patterns that might signal underlying factors or missed diagnoses. By understanding how a patient has responded to past treatments and their unique psychiatric landscape, practitioners can avoid a one-size-fits-all approach, tailoring interventions to meet the patient's specific needs.

Lifestyle Assessment

Finally, a **lifestyle assessment** is a cornerstone of functional psychiatry, as lifestyle factors often play a major role in mental health. Diet can influence neurotransmitter levels, sleep impacts cognitive function and mood stability, and exercise is known to release endorphins and improve resilience to stress. Stress management is equally important, as chronic stress can elevate cortisol and exacerbate mental health symptoms. By evaluating these lifestyle components, practitioners can identify imbalances that may be contributing to psychiatric symptoms. For instance, a patient with a diet high in processed foods and low in essential nutrients may benefit from dietary adjustments to support brain function and emotional regulation. This holistic view of lifestyle provides actionable insights that can improve mental health outcomes in lasting, meaningful ways.

A comprehensive functional assessment brings together these diverse components—holistic evaluation, physical markers, mental health history, and lifestyle factors—offering a detailed, personalized picture of a patient's mental health. This approach aims to identify and address the root causes of psychiatric symptoms, setting the stage for sustainable mental well-being.

Key Biological and Genetic Markers in Diagnosis

Biological and genetic factors play a critical role in shaping mental health, often influencing how symptoms develop, persist, or respond to treatment. In functional psychiatry, identifying these factors helps create a more accurate, personalized diagnostic picture. Understanding the underlying **genetic predispositions**, **biochemical imbalances**, and **inflammatory markers** provides insights into the root causes of mental health issues, guiding effective interventions. This section explores these markers in detail, illustrating their relevance in psychiatric assessment and treatment.

Genetic Predispositions

Genetic predispositions can significantly impact an individual's vulnerability to mental health conditions. Genes interact with lifestyle and environmental factors to either enhance resilience or increase susceptibility to psychiatric disorders. For example, variations in the **MTHFR gene** can affect the body's ability to metabolize folate, which is essential for neurotransmitter production. Individuals with certain MTHFR variants may be more prone to depression or anxiety due to impaired methylation, a biochemical process critical for mental and physical health. Another relevant marker is the **COMT enzyme**, which influences dopamine breakdown. Variations in the COMT gene can affect dopamine levels in the brain, impacting cognitive function, emotional regulation, and stress response. Identifying these genetic factors provides a deeper understanding of a patient's mental health profile, offering clues about potential underlying issues that traditional diagnostic methods might overlook. Genetic testing for these markers helps functional psychiatry tailor interventions, including nutritional supplementation and lifestyle modifications, to support optimal mental health.

Biochemical Imbalances

Biochemical imbalances are another critical aspect of functional diagnosis, as levels of neurotransmitters and hormones directly affect mood, cognition, and behavior. **Neurotransmitters** like serotonin and dopamine play pivotal roles in mental health. Low serotonin levels, for instance, are associated with depression and anxiety, while imbalances in dopamine can lead to issues with motivation, focus, and mood regulation. Testing for neurotransmitter levels, although not always precise, can provide valuable insights into underlying biochemical factors affecting mental health. Functional psychiatry often uses these findings as part of a broader assessment, incorporating dietary adjustments or supplements to support neurotransmitter balance.

Hormonal imbalances are equally important, with **cortisol and thyroid hormones** standing out as major contributors to psychiatric symptoms. **Cortisol**, the body's primary stress hormone, affects energy levels, mood stability, and sleep quality. Chronic elevation of cortisol, often due to long-term stress, can lead to symptoms of anxiety, depression, and fatigue. Testing cortisol levels through saliva or blood tests can reveal stress-related patterns that impact mental health. **Thyroid hormones** (T3 and T4) are also essential for cognitive function and emotional stability. Hypothyroidism, a condition in which thyroid hormone levels are too low, can mimic symptoms of depression, including fatigue, low mood, and cognitive "fog." Comprehensive thyroid testing, which includes TSH, T3, and T4 levels, can identify these imbalances, enabling targeted treatments such as hormone therapy or nutritional interventions to restore balance.

Inflammation and Immune System

Chronic inflammation is increasingly recognized as a contributing factor to mental health disorders. Inflammation can disrupt neurotransmitter production, impair neuroplasticity, and contribute to symptoms like **brain fog, mood swings, and fatigue**. In functional psychiatry, markers like **C-reactive protein (CRP)** and **cytokines** are used to assess inflammation levels. Elevated CRP levels, for example, are associated with depression and anxiety. Cytokines, which are proteins released by immune cells in response to inflammation, can cross the blood-brain barrier and affect brain function, contributing to psychiatric symptoms. High cytokine levels have been linked to mood disorders and cognitive decline, making them relevant indicators for a functional psychiatric assessment.

Understanding the role of inflammation allows practitioners to address its sources, such as diet, stress, and environmental toxins, in order to reduce its impact on mental health. Anti-inflammatory interventions, which might include dietary changes, stress reduction techniques, and supplements like omega-3 fatty acids, can support mood stabilization and improve overall well-being by lowering inflammation levels in the body.

Case Example

Consider a patient diagnosed with chronic depression who, despite standard antidepressant treatment, continued to struggle with persistent fatigue and low mood. A functional assessment revealed significantly elevated CRP levels, indicating systemic inflammation likely contributing to her symptoms. By addressing this inflammation through an anti-inflammatory diet, stress management practices, and specific supplements, her depressive symptoms and fatigue gradually diminished. This case illustrates how identifying and treating underlying inflammation can lead to improvements in mental health beyond what traditional psychiatric treatment might achieve.

Through a detailed examination of genetic, biochemical, and inflammatory markers, functional psychiatry builds a diagnostic framework that reveals the biological underpinnings of mental health. By understanding these factors, practitioners can craft treatment plans tailored to each patient's unique physiological profile, supporting more effective and sustainable mental health outcomes.

The Gut-Brain Axis and Mental Health

The **gut-brain axis** is a communication network that links the central nervous system with the enteric nervous system in the gastrointestinal tract. This connection allows for a two-way flow of information between the brain and gut, heavily influencing mental health. Gut bacteria, known collectively as the **gut microbiome**, play a critical role in this process, producing neurotransmitters like serotonin and dopamine, which directly impact mood and cognitive function. Additionally, a significant portion of the body's immune system resides in the gut, meaning that gut health is closely linked to inflammatory responses that can affect brain function. When the gut is compromised—through poor diet, stress, or infections—mental health symptoms like anxiety, depression, and cognitive decline may arise, highlighting the central role of the gut-brain axis in psychiatric health.

Common Gut Health Markers

Assessing gut health involves examining various indicators, each of which can provide valuable insights into the state of the gut-brain axis. **Microbiome diversity** is a key factor, as a diverse gut microbiome is generally associated with better health outcomes, including mental resilience. Low diversity or overgrowth of certain bacteria can disrupt neurotransmitter production and immune balance, affecting mood and cognition. Another crucial marker is **gut permeability**, often referred to as "leaky gut." In a healthy gut, the intestinal lining acts as a barrier, allowing nutrients to pass through while blocking harmful substances. When this barrier is compromised, inflammatory molecules can enter the bloodstream and reach the brain, potentially contributing to psychiatric symptoms. **Digestive health markers** like short-chain fatty acids (byproducts of gut bacteria) and enzymes involved in nutrient absorption also provide insight into gut function and its impact on mental health. Together, these markers help practitioners assess the gut's influence on mental well-being.

Impact of Dysbiosis on Mental Health

Dysbiosis—an imbalance in gut bacteria—can have a profound effect on mental health, contributing to conditions such as anxiety, depression, and cognitive impairment. When harmful bacteria outnumber beneficial strains, the gut produces fewer beneficial neurotransmitters and more inflammatory compounds. For example, low levels of beneficial bacteria like Lactobacillus and Bifidobacterium have been associated with increased symptoms of depression. Dysbiosis may also lead to a heightened stress response, as certain gut bacteria influence cortisol production. By disrupting normal neurotransmitter synthesis and increasing inflammatory signals to the brain, dysbiosis can exacerbate psychiatric symptoms, creating a cycle that reinforces both poor gut health and poor mental health.

Practical Diagnostic Tools

Functional psychiatry uses several diagnostic tools to assess gut health and its potential impact on mental well-being. **Stool tests** analyze the microbiome, revealing the presence of beneficial and harmful bacteria, parasites, and yeast, as well as markers of inflammation and digestive function. These tests can provide actionable insights, helping practitioners identify imbalances or signs of dysbiosis. **Food sensitivity testing** is another useful tool, as food intolerances can cause inflammation and stress the gut lining, potentially aggravating mental health symptoms. Both of these assessments are valuable for patients with persistent psychiatric symptoms that do not respond to traditional treatments, as they can reveal underlying issues within the gut-brain axis. By addressing these gut health issues through targeted interventions like dietary adjustments, probiotics, and anti-inflammatory strategies, functional psychiatry offers a more comprehensive approach to mental health care.

Understanding and supporting the gut-brain axis allows practitioners to address psychiatric symptoms at their source, often providing relief that traditional psychiatric treatments alone may not achieve. This integrative approach emphasizes the importance of a balanced microbiome and a healthy gut, positioning gut health as a central pillar in the pursuit of sustainable mental well-being.

The Role of Inflammation in Psychiatric Disorders

Chronic inflammation has been increasingly linked to a range of psychiatric symptoms, including **brain fog, mood instability, and fatigue**. Inflammation can disrupt normal brain function by altering neurotransmitter production and impairing neuroplasticity, which is the brain's ability to adapt and form new connections. This inflammatory state can lead to heightened stress responses and worsen symptoms of depression, anxiety, and cognitive decline. Research has shown that elevated levels of inflammatory molecules can cross the blood-brain barrier, affecting brain regions involved in mood regulation and cognition. Thus, addressing chronic inflammation is essential in managing and alleviating these psychiatric symptoms.

Functional psychiatry utilizes specific **inflammatory markers** to assess and address inflammation's impact on mental health. Key markers include **C-reactive protein (CRP)**, an indicator of systemic inflammation, and **cytokines**, which are signaling proteins released by the immune system. Elevated CRP levels and pro-inflammatory cytokines are often seen in patients with depression and anxiety. **Testing for these markers** provides practitioners with valuable information about the role of inflammation in a patient's psychiatric symptoms. When elevated levels are detected, anti-inflammatory strategies, such as dietary changes, stress management, and targeted supplements, can be implemented to support mental health by reducing systemic inflammation.

Key Takeaways

A functional psychiatric diagnosis goes beyond symptoms, incorporating a **comprehensive assessment** of biological, psychological, and lifestyle factors. Key insights come from **biological markers** like genetic predispositions and inflammation, which reveal deeper causes of mental health conditions. **Gut health and inflammation** are essential areas for evaluation, offering a fuller understanding of the patient's overall mental and physical health. This approach allows practitioners to develop more accurate, individualized diagnoses that support sustainable treatment outcomes.

Action Step: Reflect on a patient who could benefit from assessing dietary habits, inflammation levels, or gut health as part of their mental health care.

Call to Action: Continue to the next chapter to learn how to transform these diagnostic insights into a personalized treatment plan.

Chapter 3: Developing an Integrative Treatment Plan

"Healing takes time, and asking for help is a courageous step."
— *Mariska Hargitay*

A woman in her forties had spent years cycling through various antidepressants and sleep medications with minimal relief. Standard treatments targeted her symptoms but never seemed to touch the underlying fatigue and low mood that defined her daily life. It was only when she received a personalized, integrative treatment plan that addressed her specific nutritional deficiencies, sleep disruptions, and chronic stress that she finally began to experience true improvement. Her progress demonstrated how a tailored approach that goes beyond symptom management can lead to profound, sustainable mental health gains.

This chapter will outline how to create an individualized treatment plan that targets root causes rather than superficial symptoms. We'll cover **key steps for crafting a personalized plan**, integrating dietary changes, lifestyle modifications, and therapeutic interventions. Practical examples will illustrate how to **prioritize treatment elements** for each patient, ensuring an approach that is both manageable and highly effective for long-term mental wellness.

Personalized Treatment Planning

Effective treatment in functional psychiatry begins with a comprehensive understanding of each patient's unique health profile. A personalized treatment plan isn't simply a checklist of standard interventions; it's a tailored approach designed to address specific underlying issues, making recovery more attainable and sustainable. This section provides a roadmap for assessing patient needs, developing clear goals, and prioritizing interventions to create a treatment plan that offers targeted support while keeping the process manageable.

Assessing Patient Needs and Priorities

The first step in crafting a personalized plan involves a detailed assessment of the patient's primary health concerns and priorities. Begin by identifying the most pressing mental health symptoms, such as anxiety, depression, or mood instability, as well as any co-occurring physical symptoms, like fatigue, digestive issues, or chronic pain. Lifestyle factors—including diet, exercise, sleep quality, and stress levels—are equally important, as these often influence and exacerbate mental health conditions. Gathering information on **biological markers**, such as inflammatory levels, thyroid function, and hormonal balance, further refines the picture, allowing for a more comprehensive understanding of what's affecting the patient's mental well-being. Engaging patients in this process helps identify areas they feel are most important to address, fostering a sense of involvement and ensuring the plan aligns with their goals.

Creating an Actionable Treatment Roadmap

Once the key health areas have been identified, the next step is to establish an actionable roadmap that translates assessment findings into specific goals. Define clear objectives for each area of focus. For instance, if sleep disruption is a prominent issue, a primary goal might be to improve sleep duration and quality through a series of sleep hygiene interventions and natural supplements. Addressing dietary deficiencies, such as low levels of B vitamins or omega-3 fatty acids, may involve adding specific foods or supplements to the patient's daily intake. Reducing stress could be approached by setting goals around mindfulness practices or relaxation exercises. For each goal, break down the interventions into simple, achievable steps. This might involve **gradual dietary changes**, introducing one or two nutrient-dense foods at a time, or implementing a structured sleep routine to help reset the patient's circadian rhythm. Clearly outlining each step makes the plan more accessible for patients, empowering them to take ownership of their progress and see tangible benefits as they advance through each stage.

Prioritizing Interventions

With a range of potential interventions identified, it's essential to prioritize them based on the patient's most immediate needs. This ensures that the plan doesn't overwhelm the patient and that critical areas are addressed first. Start by identifying the interventions likely to have the greatest impact. For example, if sleep issues are severe, focusing on sleep optimization may be the best first step, as improved rest can significantly enhance overall mood, cognitive function, and resilience to stress. If dietary habits are poor and contributing to mood instability, dietary interventions might take precedence. Functional psychiatry often emphasizes addressing **root causes**, so prioritize foundational elements like nutrition, sleep, and stress management before moving on to more specialized or complex interventions. Keeping the initial focus on the highest-impact areas helps build momentum in treatment, showing patients early results that can motivate them to stay engaged with the process.

Personalized treatment planning transforms a static list of recommendations into a dynamic, patient-centered plan designed to achieve measurable progress. By assessing each patient's unique needs, setting specific goals, and prioritizing interventions strategically, practitioners can create a roadmap for mental health recovery that's both comprehensive and manageable, setting the stage for lasting improvement.

Dietary Interventions for Mental Health

Diet is a powerful factor in mental health, affecting everything from mood and energy levels to resilience against stress. Functional psychiatry views food as more than fuel; it's a source of essential nutrients that can support or disrupt mental well-being. This section outlines the components of a mental health-focused diet, including anti-inflammatory foods and key nutrients, tips for eliminating common trigger foods, and practical steps for implementing dietary changes.

Anti-Inflammatory and Nutrient-Rich Diets

An anti-inflammatory diet is foundational for mental health, as chronic inflammation can impair brain function and exacerbate symptoms like depression and anxiety. **Leafy greens**, **berries**, and **fatty fish** are key components of this diet due to their high levels of antioxidants and omega-3 fatty acids, which reduce inflammation and support brain health. Omega-3s, found in salmon, sardines, and flaxseeds, are particularly crucial, as they play a role in maintaining cell membrane integrity and promoting the production of mood-regulating neurotransmitters.

B vitamins—especially B6, B12, and folate—are essential for brain function, as they aid in the synthesis of neurotransmitters like serotonin and dopamine. Foods rich in B vitamins include eggs, leafy greens, and whole grains. **Magnesium**, another critical nutrient, helps regulate the body's stress response and is found in nuts, seeds, and dark chocolate. Studies link low magnesium levels to increased anxiety and mood disorders, making it a priority in mental health-focused dietary plans. Including these nutrient-rich foods in a patient's diet can help create a solid foundation for improved mood and cognitive function.

Eliminating Trigger Foods

Identifying and reducing **potential food sensitivities** is also essential, as some foods can trigger inflammation or hormonal disruptions that negatively impact mental health. Common culprits include **gluten** and **dairy**, which some individuals may be sensitive to without knowing it. Gluten sensitivity, for example, has been associated with "brain fog," mood swings, and fatigue in sensitive individuals. Similarly, dairy products can provoke inflammatory responses in those who are lactose intolerant or sensitive to casein, a protein found in milk. Eliminating these foods for a few weeks and observing any changes in mood or energy can help identify problematic foods. If symptoms improve after removing these foods, they can be gradually reintroduced to determine tolerance levels or permanently avoided if symptoms recur. This approach is simple and non-invasive, yet it can significantly impact mental well-being by reducing hidden sources of inflammation and irritation.

Practical Tips for Dietary Changes

For many patients, shifting to a mental health-friendly diet can feel overwhelming, so **gradual changes** are often the most sustainable approach. Encourage patients to start with small adjustments, such as adding one or two servings of leafy greens or berries each day, or swapping a refined carbohydrate snack for a handful of nuts rich in magnesium. **Meal planning** can also support dietary changes, helping patients avoid impulsive, less healthy choices and stay consistent with their new eating habits. Introducing new foods and practices one at a time allows patients to build confidence and creates a solid foundation for further dietary improvements. Simple actions, like keeping fresh fruit accessible or preparing meals with healthy fats and colorful vegetables, can make a difference without overwhelming the patient.

Case Example

A patient experiencing mood swings and fatigue saw significant improvement after making dietary adjustments. By reducing processed foods and incorporating more anti-inflammatory choices, like fatty fish, leafy greens, and nuts, her mood became more stable, and her energy levels increased. This example highlights the transformative potential of dietary interventions as part of a comprehensive treatment plan.

Through targeted dietary interventions, functional psychiatry provides a practical and impactful way to enhance mental health. By focusing on anti-inflammatory foods, addressing food sensitivities, and making gradual changes, patients can experience lasting improvements in mood and overall mental wellness.

Optimizing Sleep and Movement

Quality sleep and regular movement are foundational for mental health, significantly impacting mood, resilience to stress, and cognitive clarity. Functional psychiatry prioritizes these factors as essential components of an integrative treatment plan, addressing the ways poor sleep and inactivity can exacerbate symptoms and hinder recovery. This section provides strategies for optimizing sleep and movement to improve mental well-being.

Sleep Optimization

Inadequate sleep can disrupt emotional regulation, increase stress levels, and contribute to symptoms of anxiety and depression. Sleep deprivation impairs the brain's ability to process and respond to emotional stimuli, leading to irritability, mood instability, and reduced cognitive function. Poor sleep also affects memory, focus, and decision-making, making it harder for patients to manage daily challenges. To improve sleep quality, establishing a **consistent sleep schedule** is key. Going to bed and waking up at the same time each day can help reset the body's circadian rhythm, enhancing sleep depth and quality.

Reducing **screen time** before bed, particularly exposure to blue light from phones, tablets, or computers, can help as well, as blue light suppresses melatonin production, the hormone that promotes sleep. Encouraging patients to create a **pre-sleep routine** can also make a difference. This might involve winding down with calming activities like reading, gentle stretching, or practicing deep breathing exercises. Small adjustments, such as maintaining a cool, dark bedroom environment, can also promote better sleep. By establishing these sleep habits, patients can often experience improvements in mood, clarity, and emotional resilience.

Exercise and Physical Activity

Regular physical activity has well-documented benefits for mental health, including improved mood, increased energy, and reduced anxiety. Exercise stimulates the release of endorphins, dopamine, and serotonin, which help regulate mood and relieve stress. **Aerobic exercise**—such as brisk walking, running, or cycling—is particularly effective for boosting mental clarity and emotional stability. Studies have shown that even moderate-intensity aerobic exercise can significantly reduce symptoms of depression and anxiety. For overall mental health, aiming for at least 150 minutes of moderate aerobic exercise per week is a reasonable goal.

Strength training can also be beneficial, as it improves physical strength and has been linked to higher self-esteem and better resilience to stress. Activities like **yoga** offer both physical and mental benefits, combining movement with breath control and mindfulness, which can improve focus, reduce tension, and enhance emotional regulation. For patients new to exercise, starting small—such as a 10-minute walk each day—can make incorporating regular activity more achievable. Gradually increasing frequency and duration helps build consistency without overwhelming the patient.

Case Example

A patient dealing with mild depression and low energy found significant relief after incorporating a consistent sleep schedule and regular physical activity. By going to bed and waking up at the same time each day, her sleep quality improved, leading to better mood stability. Additionally, she started with daily 20-minute walks and eventually added strength training twice a week. Within weeks, she noticed increased energy and a more positive outlook, demonstrating how targeted adjustments in sleep and movement can foster meaningful improvements.

Optimizing sleep and incorporating physical activity into a treatment plan provides patients with accessible, practical tools to support mental health. By addressing these elements, functional psychiatry offers patients pathways to enhanced resilience, clarity, and mood stability that are both sustainable and impactful.

Stress Management and Mindfulness Practices

Chronic stress exerts a powerful impact on mental and physical health, often contributing to anxiety, depression, and a host of physical ailments like high blood pressure and weakened immunity. Persistent stress triggers the release of cortisol, the body's primary stress hormone, which, when elevated over time, disrupts sleep, weakens emotional resilience, and affects cognitive function. Integrating stress management techniques within a treatment plan is essential for helping patients build mental resilience and reduce the negative effects of stress on both mind and body.

Mindfulness and Relaxation Techniques

Mindfulness practices are effective tools for managing stress and promoting emotional balance. Simple techniques like **deep breathing exercises** help activate the body's relaxation response, counteracting the effects of stress by lowering heart rate and calming the nervous system. **Meditation**, even for just 5–10 minutes a day, encourages a state of focus and calm, helping patients center their thoughts and gain control over anxious feelings. **Grounding techniques**, such as focusing on sensory experiences (e.g., the feeling of feet on the ground or the sensation of breathing), are practical for patients who feel overwhelmed, as they shift attention away from anxious thoughts and back to the present moment.

For beginners, introducing small, manageable strategies is key to building a sustainable mindfulness routine. Encourage patients to start by practicing breathing exercises or a brief meditation each morning or during a stressful moment in the day. Over time, they can extend these practices as they grow more comfortable, gradually incorporating mindfulness into other areas of daily life, like mindful eating or walking.

Case Study

A patient with generalized anxiety disorder found mindfulness exercises transformative in managing daily stress. She began with a simple practice of deep breathing whenever she felt overwhelmed, spending just a few minutes focusing on her breath. Over time, she incorporated short meditation sessions each morning, gradually noticing improvements in her anxiety levels and overall resilience. Through these regular practices, she learned to manage her stress response more effectively, reducing her anxiety and enhancing her quality of life.

Practical Tips for Practitioners

Encourage patients to start with small, achievable mindfulness practices that fit into their routine. Simple steps—like focusing on deep breathing for two minutes each morning—can be an accessible way to introduce mindfulness, helping patients develop a foundation without feeling overwhelmed. Gradually, these small practices can be expanded, providing a pathway to lasting stress resilience and mental well-being.

Incorporating stress management and mindfulness into a treatment plan equips patients with lifelong tools for emotional regulation, improving mental health outcomes and enhancing their ability to cope with daily challenges.

Key Takeaways

A personalized, integrative approach to mental health creates more effective treatment plans by addressing each patient's unique circumstances and needs. Incorporating **diet, sleep, exercise, and stress management** provides a strong foundation for improving mental well-being. Implementing **simple, gradual changes** helps patients build sustainable habits without feeling overwhelmed, supporting long-term mental health and resilience.

Action Step: Begin designing a basic treatment plan for a current patient, incorporating one lifestyle change—such as diet, sleep, exercise, or stress management—that could benefit their mental health.

Call to Action: Continue to the next chapter to explore therapeutic techniques that complement and enhance integrative treatment plans.

Chapter 4: Integrating Therapeutic Techniques in Functional Psychiatry

"The mind has great influence over the body, and maladies often have their origin there."
— *Molière*

A patient struggling with chronic anxiety and insomnia had tried various medications and lifestyle changes with only limited success. It wasn't until her treatment incorporated cognitive-behavioral therapy (CBT) and regular mindfulness practices that her mental health began to stabilize. The combination of structured therapeutic techniques with functional lifestyle adjustments allowed her to build emotional resilience, manage stress, and finally experience restful sleep. This case highlights how integrating specific therapeutic approaches within a functional framework can elevate patient outcomes, addressing root causes while offering practical tools for lasting mental health improvement.

This chapter examines how **therapeutic techniques like CBT, mind-body practices, biofeedback, and mindful medication management** can enhance a functional psychiatry treatment plan. By blending these therapies with holistic and lifestyle interventions, practitioners can offer comprehensive, personalized care that targets both immediate symptoms and the underlying drivers of mental health issues.

Cognitive and Behavioral Interventions

Cognitive and behavioral therapies offer effective, structured approaches that align well with functional psychiatry's goal of addressing root causes and creating sustainable mental health improvements. Techniques like Cognitive-Behavioral Therapy (CBT), Dialectical Behavior Therapy (DBT), and Acceptance and Commitment Therapy (ACT) equip patients with tools to understand and reshape their thought patterns, regulate emotions, and build resilience. For individuals dealing with anxiety, depression, or trauma, these therapies provide a foundation for transforming mental and emotional responses in ways that complement lifestyle and biological interventions.

Overview of Cognitive-Behavioral Therapy (CBT)

Cognitive-Behavioral Therapy (CBT) is a well-researched approach that focuses on identifying and modifying **maladaptive thought patterns and behaviors** that negatively impact mental health. The underlying principle of CBT is that thoughts, feelings, and behaviors are interconnected, and by restructuring distorted thoughts, patients can shift their emotional responses and actions. In practice, CBT involves recognizing automatic negative thoughts, challenging their validity, and replacing them with healthier, balanced perspectives.

CBT is highly adaptable and works well in conjunction with functional methods. For example, CBT's emphasis on **self-awareness and thought restructuring** helps patients make the mental shift necessary to fully engage in lifestyle interventions, such as dietary changes or sleep improvement. Patients learn to recognize how poor sleep, for instance, might influence negative thinking patterns or heightened anxiety, creating a cycle. By addressing both thought patterns and lifestyle factors, CBT becomes an integral part of a holistic treatment plan, supporting sustainable mental health improvements.

Dialectical Behavior Therapy (DBT) and Acceptance and Commitment Therapy (ACT)

Dialectical Behavior Therapy (DBT) and Acceptance and Commitment Therapy (ACT) are therapeutic approaches that build on CBT principles with additional focus areas. DBT, initially developed for borderline personality disorder, has proven effective in treating a range of mental health conditions. It focuses on **emotional regulation, distress tolerance, and interpersonal effectiveness**. Patients learn coping skills to manage intense emotions, enabling them to respond more adaptively to stressors. This makes DBT a powerful tool for individuals with high emotional reactivity or difficulty regulating stress, allowing them to gain control over reactions that might otherwise undermine their progress in other areas, such as lifestyle adjustments or therapeutic goals.

ACT, on the other hand, encourages **acceptance of difficult thoughts and emotions rather than resisting them**. It emphasizes mindfulness and committing to actions aligned with personal values. ACT helps patients create a new relationship with their thoughts, viewing them without judgment and reducing the impact of distressing emotions. This approach is particularly helpful for patients dealing with chronic anxiety or trauma, as it teaches them to live with uncomfortable emotions rather than avoid or react to them. Integrating ACT within a functional framework allows patients to focus on lifestyle changes without becoming discouraged by negative thoughts or momentary setbacks.

Case Study

A patient with generalized anxiety found a combined approach using CBT and lifestyle adjustments highly effective. Through CBT, she recognized how her catastrophic thinking patterns heightened her anxiety. By reframing these thoughts, along with improving her sleep and diet, she noticed a marked reduction in her anxiety symptoms. Regular practice of CBT techniques, alongside these lifestyle changes, helped her sustain these improvements, demonstrating the effectiveness of combining cognitive restructuring with functional interventions.

Cognitive and behavioral therapies like CBT, DBT, and ACT play a critical role in a functional psychiatry treatment plan, equipping patients with practical tools to reshape their mental and emotional responses. These therapies work hand-in-hand with lifestyle and biological interventions, creating a comprehensive approach to mental health that empowers patients to achieve lasting change.

Mind-Body Techniques

Mind-body techniques are foundational in functional psychiatry, bridging the gap between physical and mental health to support relaxation, focus, and emotional regulation. Practices like mindfulness, meditation, yoga, and tai chi help patients cultivate self-awareness, reduce stress, and manage difficult emotions more effectively. By addressing the body and mind simultaneously, these techniques create a strong foundation for mental health improvement, enhancing the effects of other treatments in a functional plan.

Introduction to Mind-Body Techniques

Mind-body practices are particularly effective because they work on both psychological and physiological levels, reducing the impact of chronic stress while fostering emotional resilience. Techniques like mindfulness and yoga promote relaxation and help regulate the nervous system, which is often overactivated in individuals facing mental health challenges. Regular practice increases **mindfulness and self-compassion**, empowering patients to approach their thoughts and emotions without judgment. This approach helps patients respond to stressors rather than react impulsively, leading to a more balanced emotional state. Functional psychiatry integrates these practices to improve overall mental health outcomes, creating a more comprehensive treatment that addresses both internal and external influences on mental well-being.

Mindfulness and Meditation

Mindfulness is the practice of observing thoughts and sensations without judgment, fostering a sense of calm and focus in the present moment. **Meditation**, closely related, involves structured mental exercises to promote relaxation and focus. Both mindfulness and meditation have shown significant benefits in managing **anxiety, depression, and stress**, as they help patients cultivate a state of awareness that prevents them from becoming overwhelmed by their thoughts. Studies show that mindfulness and meditation decrease stress hormone levels, increase serotonin production, and improve neural pathways related to emotional regulation.

Patients can benefit from simple mindfulness techniques that are easy to incorporate into daily life. **Breathing exercises**, for example, involve taking slow, deep breaths to calm the nervous system and alleviate anxiety. Patients can also use **body scans**, a practice in which they mentally "scan" each body part, releasing tension as they go. These exercises can be done in just a few minutes and offer immediate relief from stress. Encouraging patients to start with brief sessions helps establish a consistent routine, building a habit that can lead to long-term mental health improvements.

Yoga and Tai Chi

Yoga and tai chi are movement-based practices that combine physical exercise with mindfulness, supporting both physical relaxation and mental clarity. **Yoga** incorporates deep breathing, stretching, and meditation to help release physical tension and calm the mind. Practicing yoga regularly has been shown to decrease symptoms of anxiety and depression, as well as improve sleep quality. **Tai chi**, a form of moving meditation that originated in China, uses slow, deliberate movements to foster relaxation and focus, balancing energy in the body. Both practices help patients become more in tune with their bodies, releasing stored tension that may exacerbate mental health issues.

Case Study

A patient with PTSD found significant improvement by combining yoga and meditation with therapy. The physical movement in yoga allowed her to release tension and focus on the present, while meditation provided mental grounding. This integrated approach stabilized her mood and reduced PTSD symptoms, illustrating the powerful impact of mind-body techniques in a holistic treatment plan.

Mind-body practices like mindfulness, meditation, yoga, and tai chi offer patients effective tools for managing stress and improving emotional well-being. By promoting relaxation, focus, and self-compassion, these techniques align well with functional psychiatry's commitment to addressing mental health in a comprehensive, integrative way.

Biofeedback and Neurofeedback

Biofeedback and **neurofeedback** are powerful tools for managing stress, anxiety, and trauma by helping patients gain control over their physiological responses. Biofeedback teaches individuals to regulate functions like **heart rate, muscle tension, and skin temperature**, which are often impacted by stress and emotional disturbances. Through sensors attached to the body, patients receive real-time feedback on these physiological processes, enabling them to adjust and calm their responses consciously. Neurofeedback, a specialized form of biofeedback, targets **brainwave activity** to help individuals modulate mental states. Neurofeedback has shown effectiveness in treating conditions like **ADHD, anxiety, and PTSD** by training patients to maintain optimal brainwave patterns for focus and relaxation.

These techniques align well with functional psychiatry's integrative approach, as they empower patients to understand and manage their responses to stressors. By learning to self-regulate, patients can reduce the frequency and severity of symptoms, complementing other therapeutic interventions, lifestyle adjustments, and dietary changes. Neurofeedback, specifically, allows patients to reshape their brain's activity, offering a non-invasive, drug-free method for enhancing cognitive function and emotional regulation.

Practical Applications

Biofeedback can be seamlessly integrated into a functional treatment plan, especially for patients with high anxiety or those who struggle with emotional reactivity. For example, **controlled breathing exercises** guided by biofeedback can lower heart rate and blood pressure, immediately reducing the physical symptoms of anxiety. Patients learn to practice these techniques independently, using breathing and muscle relaxation to manage stress before it escalates. Similarly, neurofeedback sessions can help patients, particularly those with ADHD or PTSD, practice and reinforce brainwave patterns that support focus, calmness, and resilience to stress. Over time, this training enables patients to naturally maintain these regulated states, even in challenging situations.

Case Study

A young adult with ADHD experienced significant improvements in focus and emotional regulation after undergoing neurofeedback sessions. By combining neurofeedback training with lifestyle modifications—such as a structured sleep schedule and a nutrient-rich diet tailored to his needs—he developed better self-control and concentration. Neurofeedback enabled him to strengthen brainwave patterns associated with attention, which, along with lifestyle adjustments, helped reduce the need for medication and improved his academic and social performance.

Biofeedback and neurofeedback empower patients with skills to regulate their physiological and mental states, providing valuable support for managing complex mental health conditions. As part of a functional psychiatry treatment plan, these techniques enhance resilience, self-awareness, and control, complementing other therapies and lifestyle changes to create a well-rounded approach to mental health.

Using Psychopharmacology with Functional Methods

In functional psychiatry, the goal is to address root causes and use **medication only when necessary**. While the emphasis remains on lifestyle, nutritional, and therapeutic interventions, medication plays a crucial role in stabilizing patients with severe symptoms. For conditions such as severe depression, bipolar disorder, or acute anxiety, medication can provide immediate relief, allowing patients to reach a level of functionality where they can engage with other aspects of treatment. In these cases, medications like antidepressants, mood stabilizers, or anxiolytics can be essential tools that support patients through periods of intense symptomatology, providing a foundation upon which functional treatments can build.

Integrating Medication with Holistic Approaches

Medication, when used judiciously, can be effectively combined with **holistic treatments** to create a balanced and sustainable treatment plan. By incorporating lifestyle modifications, nutritional adjustments, and therapeutic techniques alongside medication, patients benefit from a more comprehensive approach. For example, antidepressants can be paired with **sleep optimization practices** to improve mood stability, while **anti-inflammatory diets** and **supplements** like omega-3s and magnesium can enhance brain health and reduce medication side effects. Psychotherapy, especially cognitive-behavioral therapy (CBT) and mindfulness practices, can be integrated to help patients develop emotional regulation and coping skills. This combination allows medication to serve as a stabilizing force while functional interventions work on addressing underlying causes, ultimately helping patients reduce their reliance on medication as their overall health improves.

Case Study

A patient with severe depression struggled to function daily, despite previous attempts at lifestyle changes and therapy alone. After starting a low dose of antidepressants, her symptoms stabilized enough for her to engage in other treatments. She began working with her therapist on CBT to manage negative thought patterns and incorporated dietary changes, adding nutrient-dense foods high in omega-3s and B vitamins. Regular sleep routines and gentle exercise helped to maintain energy and improve her mood. Over time, the functional interventions strengthened her mental health, allowing for a gradual reduction in medication dosage under her psychiatrist's guidance.

Integrating psychopharmacology with functional methods provides a **balanced, holistic treatment** for patients facing severe mental health challenges. This approach respects the role of medication for immediate symptom management while prioritizing functional interventions that address long-term well-being, creating a foundation for sustainable mental health improvements.

Key Takeaways

Cognitive and behavioral therapies, mind-body practices, and biofeedback are powerful tools within functional psychiatry, enhancing mental health through holistic support. Combining these therapeutic techniques with lifestyle and biological adjustments fosters sustainable mental health improvements. Medication, when necessary, can be integrated to provide immediate symptom relief while functional methods address root causes, creating a balanced, comprehensive treatment plan.

Action Step: Identify one therapeutic technique—such as CBT or mindfulness—that could be incorporated with functional methods in current practice.

Call to Action: Proceed to the next chapter to learn how to implement functional psychiatry practically within a clinical setting, maximizing patient outcomes.

Chapter 5: Implementing Functional Psychiatry in Clinical Practice

"Alone we can do so little; together we can do so much." — Helen Keller

A mental health professional who had relied on traditional treatment methods began introducing functional elements—first small adjustments, then more substantial changes. Over time, patients not only found relief from immediate symptoms but reported broader improvements in well-being, resilience, and satisfaction with their treatment. This shift to a functional approach, rooted in collaboration and tailored care, brought new depth to her practice, enhancing patient outcomes by addressing underlying causes and involving patients actively in their own recovery.

This chapter outlines **practical steps for transitioning to a functional psychiatry model**, including strategies for building collaborative networks and establishing referral systems for comprehensive care. It also covers essential techniques for **effective patient communication and engagement**, along with methods for tracking progress to ensure consistent, sustainable improvement. These steps will guide practitioners in creating a practice that offers holistic, well-rounded mental health care, strengthening the foundation for long-term patient success.

Building a Functional Psychiatry Practice

Shifting from traditional psychiatry to a functional model involves a thoughtful, phased approach. Transitioning gradually allows practitioners to incorporate new elements without overwhelming themselves or their patients. This section outlines steps to make the shift, create a resource-rich environment, and set clear expectations to engage patients effectively in this collaborative approach.

Steps to Transition to Functional Psychiatry

Transitioning to functional psychiatry starts with incremental changes that can easily be integrated into an existing practice. Begin by introducing **small lifestyle assessments**—like asking about diet, sleep, and stress levels—to gain a broader understanding of patients' overall health. These conversations pave the way for larger functional elements, such as detailed nutritional plans or integrative mental health interventions. Over time, practitioners can layer on **additional functional components**, including personalized diagnostic tools, gut health assessments, and mindfulness practices tailored to individual needs.

Ongoing education is essential to support this shift. Training in **functional medicine principles** helps practitioners develop the skills to assess and address root causes of psychiatric symptoms. Certifications in areas like nutrition, mind-body medicine, or integrative psychiatry provide a deeper understanding of these complementary practices. Resources such as the **Institute for Functional Medicine (IFM)** and courses from organizations like the **Academy of Integrative Health & Medicine (AIHM)** offer structured programs and certifications to build proficiency. Attending conferences or joining professional networks focused on functional and integrative psychiatry further enhances expertise and keeps practitioners informed about new developments and evidence-based practices.

Creating a Resource-Rich Environment

Establishing a resource-rich environment is key to supporting functional psychiatry. Essential resources include **tools for functional assessments**, such as lab tests for inflammation markers, nutrient deficiencies, and hormone levels. Handouts and educational materials on **dietary and lifestyle changes** are also valuable, providing patients with easy-to-follow guidelines for optimizing sleep, managing stress, and incorporating exercise. Having **guides on mind-body practices** like mindfulness, meditation, and yoga makes it easier to introduce these techniques as part of a comprehensive treatment plan.

Consider building a small library or digital repository where patients can access articles, recipes, and videos related to their treatment goals. Patient engagement tools, like meal planners and symptom trackers, are also useful additions, helping individuals stay proactive in their own care. This resource-rich environment reinforces the integrative approach, giving patients practical tools and information that complement the therapeutic process.

Setting Patient Expectations

Introducing patients to the functional psychiatry model requires clear, open communication. Start by explaining that this approach addresses **underlying causes rather than symptoms alone**, which can lead to lasting improvements in mental health. Emphasize that functional psychiatry is a **collaborative process**—patients are active participants in their treatment and may need to adopt lifestyle changes or complete tasks outside of therapy sessions, like maintaining a food journal or practicing mindfulness.

Discuss the **long-term benefits** of this approach, such as reduced reliance on medication, increased resilience, and better physical health, which often positively impacts mental well-being. Setting realistic expectations also means explaining that results may take time; unlike symptom-focused treatments, functional psychiatry often requires a few weeks or months for patients to notice significant improvements. By positioning the approach as an investment in their health, practitioners can foster patient buy-in and commitment to the treatment process, helping them understand that each step brings them closer to sustainable mental health.

The Multidisciplinary Approach in Action

Building a network of complementary health professionals is essential for a functional psychiatry practice. This collaborative model allows practitioners to address the many facets of a patient's mental and physical health, ensuring that no critical element is overlooked. A well-rounded network might include **nutritionists or dietitians** for dietary support, **physical therapists** for movement and rehabilitation, and **mindfulness practitioners** for stress reduction and emotional balance. Each professional brings specialized knowledge that, combined with functional psychiatry, creates a more comprehensive approach to mental health.

Working with Other Health Professionals

Different specialists play distinct roles in supporting mental health from a functional perspective. **Dietitians and nutritionists** offer personalized nutrition plans that can address deficiencies impacting mood and cognition, such as low levels of omega-3s, B vitamins, and magnesium. They can also guide patients in managing blood sugar levels and food sensitivities, which are crucial for mental stability. **Physical therapists** help patients incorporate movement into their lives, which not only improves physical function but also reduces symptoms of anxiety and depression through regular exercise. **Counselors and therapists**, especially those trained in CBT or DBT, provide structured support for addressing trauma, developing coping skills, and managing thought patterns.

Establishing and maintaining these professional relationships requires active communication and collaboration. Schedule **regular check-ins** with these specialists to discuss patient progress and share relevant insights. Using secure communication platforms, such as encrypted emails or electronic health records (EHRs) designed for shared access, ensures that all team members are informed and aligned in their treatment approach. Clear communication channels allow each professional to work within their area of expertise while aligning their efforts with the broader goals of the functional treatment plan.

Creating Referral Networks

A reliable referral network enhances a functional psychiatry practice by providing patients with access to diverse expertise and support. When selecting professionals to refer to, look for those who understand and support the principles of functional medicine, particularly those who focus on **root causes and integrative approaches**. Meeting with potential collaborators to discuss their approach and philosophy can ensure that they are a good fit. Review credentials, experience, and specializations that are relevant to mental health, such as a dietitian experienced in mood disorders or a physical therapist who uses holistic practices.

Additionally, having a network of vetted professionals gives patients confidence in the quality of their care. Functional psychiatry benefits from this holistic approach, as patients are more likely to experience improved outcomes when they receive support tailored to all aspects of their health.

Case Study

A patient with chronic anxiety and digestive issues benefited significantly from an integrative team approach. Initially, she worked with her psychiatrist on CBT, while a nutritionist helped address her gut health with a tailored anti-inflammatory diet. When digestive issues improved, her anxiety levels decreased, and she could focus more effectively during therapy sessions. A physical therapist introduced gentle yoga exercises to reduce tension, which further alleviated her anxiety. This team-based approach allowed her to achieve substantial, lasting improvements by addressing her mental and physical health simultaneously.

A multidisciplinary network is a cornerstone of functional psychiatry, enriching the treatment process by integrating complementary expertise. By collaborating with nutritionists, physical therapists, and mindfulness practitioners, functional psychiatrists can offer patients comprehensive, well-rounded care that addresses all aspects of their well-being, leading to more sustainable outcomes.

Patient Communication and Engagement

Effective communication is essential in functional psychiatry, as it helps patients understand the benefits of this holistic approach and builds the trust needed for long-term engagement. Patients may be new to the concept of functional psychiatry, so it's important to convey how this approach empowers them to address the root causes of mental health challenges. This section provides strategies for communicating the functional model's value, encouraging active patient involvement, and fostering adherence through small, achievable goals.

Explaining the Functional Approach

Patients need a clear understanding of how functional psychiatry differs from traditional methods. Emphasize that this approach goes beyond symptom management by addressing underlying issues through **lifestyle, nutrition, and mental health interventions**. Explain the **patient-centered** nature of the model, highlighting how it's tailored to each individual's unique circumstances and health profile. Be prepared to address common questions, such as the time commitment required or the extent of lifestyle changes involved. Reassure patients that while functional psychiatry requires active participation, the benefits are typically more sustainable and transformative.

It's helpful to frame lifestyle changes as gradual, emphasizing that success comes from steady, incremental steps rather than drastic shifts. Share examples of how small changes can lead to big improvements over time, helping patients feel motivated and less intimidated by the prospect of altering their routines.

Encouraging Patient Participation

Engaging patients actively in their care is crucial for successful outcomes. In functional psychiatry, patients play a direct role in shaping their health through lifestyle and behavioral changes. Encourage them to set small, realistic goals that are both manageable and personally meaningful. For instance, if a patient's goal is to improve energy levels, they might start with a single dietary adjustment, such as including a nutrient-dense breakfast each day. As patients reach these smaller milestones, they often feel more confident and motivated to make further adjustments.

To sustain engagement, provide regular positive reinforcement and check-ins on their progress. This collaborative approach reinforces a sense of accountability and partnership, which can deepen their commitment to the treatment plan and increase adherence to new habits.

Case Example

A patient with chronic fatigue initially hesitated to make dietary changes, concerned about the time and effort involved. After discussing the benefits and starting with a simple goal—replacing sugary snacks with healthier options—she noticed a gradual increase in energy. With each success, she became more invested in her treatment, expanding her goals to include regular meal planning and improving sleep. Her commitment to small steps led to lasting lifestyle changes and marked improvements in her symptoms.

Tracking Progress and Adjusting Treatment Plans

Monitoring patient progress is critical to ensure that a functional treatment plan remains effective and responsive to evolving needs. Tracking allows practitioners to measure improvement across various health markers and provides insights on when adjustments may be necessary. This section outlines methods for observing progress, recognizing the need for change, and maintaining thorough documentation.

Monitoring Key Indicators of Progress

Functional psychiatry tracks a wide range of **indicators**, from mood stability and energy levels to physical symptoms and lifestyle habits. Improvements in sleep quality, dietary adherence, stress resilience, and emotional regulation are also relevant markers. Patient journals, standardized questionnaires, and progress notes are valuable tools for monitoring these indicators, as they provide measurable data over time. For example, mood charts can track daily emotional fluctuations, while energy and symptom journals help identify patterns in physical and mental well-being. These tools allow both the practitioner and patient to observe progress objectively and identify any areas that may need additional support.

When to Reevaluate and Adjust Treatment

Treatment plans in functional psychiatry are designed to be flexible, adapting to the patient's needs as they evolve. Regular evaluations help determine whether the current interventions are effective or if adjustments are required. If progress stalls or new symptoms emerge, it may be necessary to revisit aspects of the treatment, such as introducing new dietary changes, modifying exercise routines, or adjusting therapeutic techniques. Encourage patients to communicate openly about any changes they notice, positive or negative, to facilitate timely adjustments. This patient-responsive approach ensures that treatment remains aligned with their current health goals, enhancing overall effectiveness.

Tools for Tracking and Documentation

Maintaining accurate records is essential for tracking progress and making informed adjustments. Digital tools like EHR systems, secure note-taking apps, and progress-tracking software streamline this process and ensure data is accessible and organized. For patient engagement, apps that allow them to log symptoms, track habits, or record mood changes in real time can be particularly useful. Thorough documentation not only enhances care quality but also provides a structured view of the patient's journey, offering insights that guide further treatment adaptations.

Tracking and adjusting treatment plans support a functional psychiatry model that remains adaptable and patient-centered, ensuring patients experience continuous, meaningful improvements in their mental and physical health.

Key Takeaways

Implementing functional psychiatry is a step-by-step process that relies on comprehensive resources, patient education, and ongoing support. A **multidisciplinary network** is invaluable, allowing for holistic, well-rounded care that addresses all aspects of patient health. Clear communication, active patient engagement, and consistent progress tracking are critical for achieving long-term, sustainable results.

Action Step: Identify one area in your practice to enhance with functional psychiatry principles, whether by building a referral network or integrating a new patient-tracking tool.

Call to Action: Continue exploring functional psychiatry to deepen its impact on your practice and patient outcomes, embracing its potential for transformative change.

Conclusion

"Health is a state of complete harmony of the body, mind, and spirit."
— B.K.S. Iyengar

Functional psychiatry stands as a patient-centered, integrative approach that prioritizes the **mind-body connection** and addresses mental health issues at their root. Throughout this book, we've explored how the functional model identifies underlying causes—such as nutritional deficiencies, inflammation, and lifestyle factors—to create personalized, holistic treatment plans. Unlike conventional approaches that may focus primarily on symptom relief, functional psychiatry embraces the **whole person**, creating lasting change by balancing biological, psychological, and environmental factors.

The integrative diagnostic and treatment processes lie at the heart of this model, involving tools that assess everything from genetic markers and gut health to stress resilience. These comprehensive assessments form the basis of **individualized treatment plans** that blend lifestyle adjustments, nutritional interventions, mind-body practices, and when necessary, carefully managed medication. Above all, functional psychiatry emphasizes an **empowered, collaborative approach** where patients play an active role in their own healing, fostering long-term resilience and mental wellness.

Functional psychiatry's holistic approach has shown **remarkable effects on mental health outcomes**, offering patients sustainable relief from conditions like anxiety, depression, and chronic stress. By targeting root causes, it not only alleviates symptoms but also builds a foundation for greater psychological resilience and overall well-being. Patients often report improvements that go beyond mental health, including enhanced energy levels, better sleep, and reduced physical ailments, underscoring the interconnected nature of mind and body.

The focus on **whole-person healing** brings attention to all aspects of patients' lives, creating a more rounded picture of health. By integrating tools that address diet, movement, stress, and emotional health, functional psychiatry offers more than just treatment; it provides a pathway to lasting wellness. Patients feel genuinely cared for and understood, often experiencing mental health in a new light—one that empowers them to actively participate in their care. This empowerment translates into **increased adherence** to treatment recommendations, greater patient satisfaction, and overall improved quality of life.

As with any transformative approach, functional psychiatry comes with its own set of challenges. Practitioners may face **resistance from traditional models**, as well as logistical hurdles like limited access to functional training programs or specialized diagnostic tools. Shifting from conventional psychiatry to a functional model requires time, resources, and a commitment to ongoing learning, which can be demanding, especially in smaller practices.

Yet, the field is also ripe with **emerging opportunities**. The rise in patient demand for integrative and holistic mental health options has spurred a growing body of research, new resources, and expanded professional support. As functional psychiatry gains visibility, practitioners have a unique opportunity to lead the movement toward more effective, patient-centered mental health care. Advocacy plays a crucial role here: by sharing positive outcomes, educating patients, and engaging with other professionals, readers can help increase acceptance of functional psychiatry and build networks that strengthen the field's impact.

To continue building a functional psychiatry practice, practitioners can begin with **ongoing education** in core principles. Courses, certifications, and professional conferences are valuable for deepening expertise and staying current with evidence-based practices. The **Institute for Functional Medicine** and organizations focused on integrative health offer structured learning options that cover diagnostics, therapeutic techniques, and specialized interventions that can enrich clinical practice.

Networking and collaboration are equally important in this field, as they provide a support system for shared knowledge, referrals, and resources. Connecting with other functional and integrative health professionals—such as nutritionists, physical therapists, and counselors—enhances the range of care available to patients, allowing for a truly multidisciplinary approach. Engaging in professional groups and forums can also provide insights into best practices and innovative treatment methods.

Starting with small, meaningful changes is key to **building a patient-centered practice**. Practitioners might begin by offering lifestyle assessments or mindfulness practices in their sessions, setting the stage for deeper functional interventions as patients grow comfortable with the model. Additionally, setting clear personal and professional goals helps in tracking progress. For instance, a practitioner might aim to offer one new diagnostic tool or treatment option each quarter, ensuring that the practice evolves without overwhelming patients or staff.

Functional psychiatry holds the potential to transform mental health care into a field that is not only therapeutic but also compassionate and comprehensive. By addressing patients holistically and emphasizing the harmony of body, mind, and spirit, practitioners contribute to a vision of mental health that is both empowering and enduring. Functional psychiatry isn't just about treating symptoms—it's about fostering resilience, promoting self-care, and empowering patients to take charge of their well-being.

The future of psychiatry depends on practitioners who are willing to **lead with empathy and innovation**. Those who adopt functional psychiatry play a pivotal role in shaping a field that values each patient as a whole person, honoring their unique experiences and needs. The functional approach goes beyond temporary relief, creating a path to meaningful, long-term health.

As readers take this work forward, they carry the potential to make an incredible difference—one patient at a time. Through commitment to functional psychiatry, practitioners can offer a model of care that transforms lives, providing patients with the tools and support they need to achieve true wellness.

Explore, learn, and grow within the realm of functional psychiatry, committing to a practice that brings true harmony to patients' lives. Each step taken toward a holistic approach is a step toward a brighter future for mental health care.

www.ingramcontent.com/pod-product-compliance
Lightning Source LLC
Chambersburg PA
CBHW050259220526
45465CB00002B/744